Overstimulated

Coping with Sensory Overload as an Adult: A Practical Guide to Calm, Clarity, and Nervous System Recovery

Eric Foreman

Cipher Hayes Books

Contents

Before You Begin

A little gift from us to you

As a thank you for picking up this book, we'd love to offer you a free seasonal title and other heartfelt reads throughout the year.

Download your free book and check for new releases here:
www.cipherhayesbooks.com/download

We update this page often, so feel free to return anytime.

Happy reading—
and may this season bring you warmth, memory, and peace.

INTRODUCTION

Why You Feel So Overwhelmed—and Why It's
Not Your Fault

If you've ever found yourself emotionally drained after a
day of bright lights, loud conversations, scrolling
notifications, or even the fabric of your clothes rubbing the
wrong way—you're not alone. More adults than ever are
struggling with sensory overload, but most don't know
what to call it, let alone how to cope with it. Instead, they're
told they're too sensitive, too reactive, or too dramatic.

This book exists to challenge that narrative.

Sensory overload is not a personality flaw. It is a
physiological response to a world that is louder, faster,
brighter, and more demanding than ever before. And for
some people—especially those who are highly sensitive,
neurodivergent, trauma survivors, or living with chronic
anxiety—those daily stimuli don't just feel unpleasant.
They feel impossible.

As adults, we're expected to push through discomfort.
We're taught to suppress our needs in favor of productivity.
We overcommit, stay plugged in, and minimize our
symptoms because that's what we think we're supposed to
do. But this often leads to burnout, mental fatigue,

emotional shutdowns, and in some cases, a complete disconnection from our own needs.

This book is your guide back to yourself.

Here, we'll explore what sensory overload really is—from the science of your nervous system to the practical realities of navigating crowded offices, busy households, and digital overstimulation. You'll learn how to identify your unique triggers, develop calming strategies, and build a life that supports your sensory well-being rather than punishing it.

You'll also learn how to:

- Create physical and emotional environments that reduce overwhelm
- Set healthy boundaries with people and technology
- Calm your body in the middle of a sensory episode
- Redesign your routines around rest and regulation
- Reframe your sensitivity as a strength, not a weakness

This is not a clinical manual, nor is it a book filled with vague advice like "just reduce stress." It's a grounded, evidence-informed, and practical companion for anyone who feels overstimulated by everyday life and wants to regain a sense of peace, control, and clarity.

Whether you've been living with this for years or you're just beginning to notice the signs, this book is designed to meet you where you are. Each chapter builds upon the last, offering not just information, but transformation.

By the end, you'll not only understand what's been happening to you—you'll know what to do about it. You'll have tools, insights, and frameworks to support yourself. And most importantly, you'll no longer feel like you have to go through it alone.

Let's begin.

CHAPTER 1: WHEN THE WORLD FEELS TOO LOUD

Understanding the Modern Landscape of Sensory Overload

You're standing in line at a busy grocery store. The lights overhead are fluorescent and sharp. There's a toddler screaming two aisles away. Music is playing over the speakers—too loud, too upbeat—and the beeping of the checkout scanner keeps repeating. Your phone buzzes with a new notification, and a stranger behind you starts talking on speakerphone. You haven't even reached the front of the line yet, but your heart is racing, your jaw is tense, and something inside you is already preparing to shut down.

If that scenario feels painfully familiar, you're not imagining it.

What you're experiencing isn't just stress. It's sensory overload—and it's something millions of adults live with every day, often without realizing what it is or why it's happening.

What Is Sensory Overload?

Sensory overload occurs when your brain is unable to effectively process and filter the amount of sensory input it's receiving. This input can be auditory (noise), visual (light or clutter), tactile (clothing textures or temperature), olfactory (smells), or even emotional (too many social cues at once). For some, even internal stimuli—such as chronic pain or an anxious racing heart—can contribute to the sensation.

In a healthy nervous system, the brain acts like a gatekeeper, filtering out non-essential information so you can focus on the task at hand. But when that gatekeeping function is compromised—or when the incoming data is simply too much—the result is a flood of stimuli with no outlet. This can trigger a range of physical, emotional, and cognitive symptoms: irritability, panic, shutdown, disorientation, nausea, fatigue, or even dissociation.

For many people, especially adults who are neurodivergent, highly sensitive, or managing unresolved trauma, the threshold for overload is lower than average. That doesn't mean you're weak. It means your nervous system is wired differently—and that wiring deserves understanding, not shame.

The Modern World Is Not Designed for Sensory Safety

Fifty years ago, an average day included long stretches of silence, less artificial light, and more time in natural environments. Today, we live in an always-on society where overstimulation is baked into the architecture of our lives. Urban noise, screen-based work, digital notifications, crowded commutes, harsh lighting, and emotional performance in social settings are now considered normal. But for someone with a sensitive sensory profile, this level of constant input is not neutral—it's exhausting.

The adult experience of sensory overload is often minimized or dismissed entirely. Children are more likely to receive occupational therapy, sensory-friendly classrooms, or calming spaces. Adults, on the other hand, are expected to self-regulate, self-diagnose, and self-soothe—all while maintaining full-time jobs, family responsibilities, and social obligations.

Many don't even have the language to describe what they're experiencing. Instead, they internalize the distress. They blame themselves for being easily irritated, anxious, or fatigued. They push through until they collapse.

The truth is, sensory overload is not a personality flaw. It's not an overreaction. It's a physiological reality, and it has solutions—once you know how to recognize it.

Recognizing the Signs

Sensory overload doesn't always announce itself with drama. In adults, it often shows up as a slow build. You might notice subtle shifts:

- A rising sense of agitation for no clear reason
- Sudden need to retreat from conversation
- A tightening in your chest or jaw
- Trouble concentrating or remembering things
- The urge to cry, lash out, or shut down
- A feeling of disconnection from your surroundings
- Feeling like you're "on edge" or "wired but tired"

These experiences are not imaginary. They're the warning signals of a nervous system under siege.

Over time, if left unaddressed, this state of constant overstimulation can lead to chronic stress, burnout, anxiety disorders, sleep disruption, and even physical illness. That's why understanding the root causes and developing sustainable coping strategies isn't a luxury—it's a necessity.

Why You Haven't Heard More About This

Sensory overload is underrepresented in adult wellness conversations for a few key reasons:

1. **It's often invisible.** There are no obvious outward signs, like a rash or broken limb.
2. **It overlaps with other conditions.** Anxiety, ADHD, autism, PTSD, and even chronic illness all share symptoms.
3. **It's culturally dismissed.** We live in a society that values endurance over sensitivity.
4. **Adults are expected to "tough it out."** There is little structural support for nervous system regulation in workplaces, cities, or even homes.

This silence creates a gap in care and understanding—a gap this book aims to close.

From Surviving to Reclaiming Control

The goal of this book is not just to describe the problem, but to give you the tools to manage it. We'll start by identifying your personal sensory profile—what overwhelms you, what calms you, and how your patterns show up in everyday life. From there, we'll work toward environmental adjustments, lifestyle shifts, emotional regulation techniques, and social strategies that allow you to function without constantly overriding your nervous system.

This is not about escaping the world. It's about learning to move through it without constantly paying the price of overstimulation.

You'll learn how to:

- Detect early warning signs before a full sensory episode hits
- Build an emergency "calm kit" for overload moments
- Set boundaries that protect your energy without guilt
- Create sensory-friendly routines at home, work, and in relationships
- Reconnect with your body, not just your thoughts

This journey begins with self-awareness, but it ends in self-empowerment.

You Are Not Alone

If you've been silently struggling, questioning why things that seem "normal" to others feel unbearable to you, this chapter is your permission to stop blaming yourself. Sensory overload is real. It is valid. And there are ways forward that don't require numbing, avoidance, or masking who you are.

You are not too much. You are not broken. You are living in a world that wasn't designed with your sensory needs in mind. But with the right understanding, tools, and support, you can reclaim peace, clarity, and control.

Let's take the next step together.

CHAPTER 2: AM I TOO SENSITIVE?

Reframing Sensitivity as Intelligence, Not a Flaw

There's a moment that almost everyone who experiences sensory overload reaches. It might come after a social event that left you inexplicably drained, or during a moment when something seemingly small—a flickering light, a scratchy sweater, a coworker's loud typing—completely unravels your composure. The thought surfaces quietly but powerfully:

"Maybe I'm just too sensitive."

You may have heard this from others too—delivered with concern, criticism, or confusion. Maybe it was said in passing by someone you love. Maybe it was said to shame or silence you. Over time, those four words begin to carry weight far beyond their size.

This chapter is about unburdening that weight. Because the truth is simple: sensitivity is not weakness. It is not fragility. It is not an error in your design. In fact, it is often a sign of profound intelligence and insight—especially when it comes to how your body, brain, and environment interact.

The Biology of Sensitivity

Let's begin by clearing up a common misconception: being "sensitive" is not just about emotional reactivity. Sensory sensitivity is a biologically rooted trait that affects how deeply your nervous system processes incoming information.

Research in neuroscience and psychology has shown that individuals with heightened sensory awareness often have increased neural activity in areas of the brain responsible for empathy, decision-making, and environmental scanning. They process more details. They notice patterns. They carry more data into each moment—and as a result, they may reach overload faster, especially in chaotic or emotionally charged environments.

This is particularly true for those who identify as **Highly Sensitive Persons (HSPs)**—a term coined by psychologist Dr. Elaine Aron. HSPs make up roughly 15–20% of the population and are characterized by:

- Deep processing of sensory and emotional input
- Strong emotional reactivity (to both joy and distress)
- Heightened empathy and intuition
- A tendency to feel overwhelmed by stimuli like loud noises, crowds, or bright lights

- A rich inner life, often marked by introspection and imagination

None of these traits are pathological. But they can become distressing if misunderstood, invalidated, or suppressed.

Overlap with Neurodivergence

It's also important to recognize that sensory sensitivity frequently overlaps with various forms of neurodivergence. Adults with **ADHD**, **Autism Spectrum Disorder (ASD)**, **Post-Traumatic Stress Disorder (PTSD)**, **Generalized Anxiety Disorder (GAD)**, and **Obsessive Compulsive Disorder (OCD)** often report intense sensory experiences.

These individuals may be:

- Startled by sudden sounds
- Unable to focus in visually cluttered environments
- Bothered by certain textures or smells
- Prone to shutdown or panic in crowded spaces
- Overwhelmed by multitasking or interruptions

Again, this does not reflect a character flaw. It reflects a nervous system tuned to detect and respond to stimuli that others may not even notice.

It's also worth noting that many adults go undiagnosed for most of their lives. If you've always felt "different," "too much," or "too easily overwhelmed," you may simply be living with a sensory processing profile that's never been named, let alone supported.

Cultural Misunderstanding and Shame

We live in a culture that prizes resilience, multitasking, and stoicism. People who move slowly, speak gently, or need silence are often labeled as fragile. This mindset has consequences—not just socially, but psychologically.

Sensitivity, in this cultural context, is treated as a liability. Children are told not to cry. Adults are expected to push through discomfort. Workplaces reward performance under pressure, not awareness of internal limits.

For sensitive adults, this can lead to chronic self-doubt. You may second-guess your reactions, dismiss your needs, or push yourself beyond your breaking point just to "keep up."

Eventually, you stop trusting your own signals.

But ignoring sensitivity doesn't make it disappear. It only leads to greater emotional dysregulation, nervous system burnout, and even physical illness over time.

Reclaiming the Narrative

To move forward, we need to rewrite the story that says sensitivity is something to fix or hide. We need to start seeing it for what it truly is: a form of *input intelligence—* your system is simply registering more data from the environment, and doing so at a deeper level.

Sensitivity can manifest in many forms:

- Being emotionally moved by art, music, or storytelling
- Noticing subtle changes in tone, expression, or mood
- Having a strong reaction to injustice or cruelty
- Feeling deeply connected to nature or animals
- Picking up on details others miss
- Needing longer recovery time after social or sensory-heavy events

These are not weaknesses. These are capacities. They require support—not suppression.

When you begin to see your sensitivity as something to respect rather than reject, your entire relationship with overstimulation can begin to shift.

Self-Reflection: What Kind of Sensitive Are You?

While every person's sensory profile is unique, there are some general patterns you may find helpful. Consider these questions as a starting point:

- Do loud environments leave you emotionally drained or physically tense?
- Are you particularly sensitive to certain smells, fabrics, or lighting conditions?
- Do you find multitasking or chaotic spaces overwhelming?
- Do you get easily startled or feel "on edge" in busy places?
- Do you struggle to focus when there's too much background noise?
- Do you feel physically or emotionally uncomfortable in crowds, parties, or open offices?
- Do you need more downtime than others after social events or busy workdays?

These questions aren't meant to diagnose—they're meant to increase self-awareness. Sensory needs vary, and they can change based on stress levels, sleep, hormones, or life circumstances. The more fluent you become in reading your own cues, the more effectively you can care for yourself.

You're Not Too Sensitive. You're Unprotected.

This chapter began with a familiar question: "Am I too sensitive?"

Let's reframe that.

Imagine someone walking through a blizzard without a coat. Would we say they're too cold? Or would we ask why they're not protected?

When you feel overwhelmed by lights, sounds, crowds, or emotional interactions, it's not because you're too sensitive. It's because your system is telling you it needs a coat—it needs buffering, regulation, and protection.

That's what this book is here to help you build.

In the coming chapters, we'll explore how to create that sensory protection on all levels: environmental, physical, emotional, and relational. You'll learn how to respond to overload early, how to advocate for your needs, and how to live in a way that honors your sensitivity instead of working against it.

For now, hold onto this truth:

You are not too sensitive. You are precisely as sensitive as you need to be to experience the world deeply, thoughtfully, and meaningfully.

Let's begin learning how to make that a strength, not a burden.

CHAPTER 3: THE TRIGGERS YOU DIDN'T SEE COMING

Learning to Recognize What's Overwhelming You Before It Breaks You

Sensory overload doesn't always arrive like a thunderclap. More often, it seeps in slowly—quietly stacking small irritations, background noise, and unacknowledged tension until something tips you over the edge. You snap at someone. You shut down. You feel an inexplicable wave of anxiety or exhaustion. And because the trigger wasn't obvious, you question your reaction or blame yourself.

What many people don't realize is that overload isn't always about a single event. It's about **accumulation**. One flickering light, on its own, might be manageable. But combine it with a tight waistband, a noisy office, an intense conversation, and a skipped lunch, and your nervous system is under siege.

In this chapter, we'll explore the everyday triggers that often go unnoticed. These are the stimuli that slowly build pressure in your body and mind, creating a baseline of discomfort that eventually turns into full-blown overwhelm.

The goal isn't to avoid life or control every environment. The goal is to develop **awareness**, so you can anticipate, buffer, and recover from sensory input before it harms your health or hijacks your mood.

Sensory Overload Is Often Layered, Not Singular

Many people look for one big trigger—one loud noise, one stressful conversation, one crowded space. But overload is rarely that simple. Instead, it's more like a **tipping point** reached after dozens of small inputs.

Think of your nervous system as a container. Every sensory input adds a drop. When that container is full, anything else—even something tiny—can cause a spill.

By identifying which drops are filling your container the fastest, you gain the power to reduce them, rearrange them, or recover from them more strategically.

Let's break down the most common (and often hidden) contributors to adult sensory overload.

1. *Noise Pollution You've Learned to Ignore*

Your brain may try to filter it out, but your nervous system still registers it. Chronic background noise is one of the most common and underestimated stressors for adults.

This includes:

- HVAC systems or refrigerator hums
- Office chatter, keyboard clacking, clicking pens
- Cars outside your window, barking dogs, sirens
- TV left on in another room
- Loud advertisements, public address systems
- High-pitched electronic tones you barely notice

Even low-level noise can increase cortisol, the stress hormone, and make it harder to focus. If you're in a place where your ears never get true silence, your system may stay in a constant state of low-grade alertness.

Micro-intervention: Try inserting intentional quiet into your day. Five minutes of silence—no music, no podcasts, no conversation—can give your nervous system a critical reset.

2. Lighting That Feels Hostile to Your Body

We've grown used to artificial lighting—LEDs, fluorescents, blue light from screens—but that adaptation comes at a cost for sensitive systems.

Problematic lighting can include:

- Flickering or buzzing fluorescent tubes
- Bright overhead office lights
- Lack of natural sunlight
- Harsh blue lighting from screens at night
- Excessive visual clutter from mixed light sources

You might not be consciously thinking, "This light is hurting me." But your body may be responding with squinting, tension, headaches, fatigue, or even agitation.

Micro-intervention: Soften your spaces. Use lamps instead of overhead lights. Try warm bulbs. Consider blue light filters on your screens, especially in the evening.

3. Visual Clutter and Disorganization

Your brain uses visual input to assess safety and focus. When your environment is visually chaotic, your system may stay in a low-level fight-or-flight state—constantly scanning for order that doesn't come.

Visual overload can stem from:

- Messy desks or countertops
- Too many tabs open on your computer
- Bright packaging and signage in stores
- Busy patterns, neon colors, fast-moving visuals
- Flashing notifications or pop-ups on digital devices

Clutter isn't just an aesthetic issue—it's neurological. For sensitive individuals, too much visual input creates cognitive noise, making it harder to concentrate or relax.

Micro-intervention: Tidy one visual field at a time. If your desk feels overwhelming, try clearing just one side. Reduce stimuli where you spend the most time.

4. Clothing and Physical Discomfort

What you wear can impact your sensory regulation in surprising ways. Textures, tightness, temperature—all of it matters.

Discomfort triggers may include:

- Tight waistbands, collars, or shoes
- Tags, seams, or rough fabrics
- Restrictive undergarments
- Synthetic fabrics that don't breathe

- Jewelry that jingles or shifts

Many people tolerate uncomfortable clothing because it looks appropriate, or because they've been told it's "just part of being an adult." But these micro-irritations can be draining, especially over long periods.

Micro-intervention: Audit your wardrobe for comfort, not just style. Notice how you feel after wearing certain outfits. Comfort is not a luxury—it's regulation.

5. Multitasking and Constant Switching

Every time you switch tasks—checking a text, scanning an email, opening a new tab—you tax your brain's executive function. Add in background noise, conversations, or deadlines, and your cognitive load skyrockets.

This is especially hard on people with ADHD or anxiety, but anyone can suffer from too much **context switching**, which fragments focus and floods the brain with unfinished loops.

Micro-intervention: Work in time blocks. Use timers. Close tabs. Give your brain one job at a time whenever possible.

6. *Digital Overload and Information Fatigue*

We consume more information in a day than previous generations absorbed in weeks. Emails, news, videos, social media, texts, pop-ups, podcasts—it's endless.

But your brain isn't a machine. It has limits.

Sensory overload from digital input can include:

- Notifications disrupting your focus
- News headlines triggering anxiety
- Social media comparisons draining emotional energy
- Decision fatigue from endless scrolling or content hopping

Micro-intervention: Practice digital boundaries. Silence notifications. Choose intentional scroll times. Take screen-free hours or mornings to recalibrate.

7. *Smell and Chemical Sensitivities*

You may not always notice smells consciously, but they can deeply impact your nervous system and mood. Sensitive individuals often report:

- Headaches from perfumes or cleaning products
- Nausea from synthetic air fresheners

- Fatigue from poor indoor air quality
- Mood changes triggered by body odor or food smells in enclosed spaces

Micro-intervention: Use unscented products when possible. Ventilate your home. Incorporate natural scents you enjoy—lavender, citrus, cedar—into your calm spaces.

8. Social and Emotional Input

Sensory overload isn't just physical—it's emotional too. You may become overloaded by the tone of a conversation, the number of people in a room, or even the unspoken tension between others.

Triggers may include:

- Group settings without a clear exit
- Phone calls when you're already mentally tired
- Being "on" for extended periods in meetings or caregiving roles
- High-emotion environments like weddings, funerals, or family gatherings

Micro-intervention: Schedule quiet time after high-social events. Let yourself decompress. It's not anti-social to recover. It's self-respect.

Reflection: What's Filling Your Cup?

Use this metaphor throughout your day: **What's filling my sensory cup right now?** Is it visual noise? Is it a tight outfit? Is it emotional labor?

Begin keeping a **Sensory Log**. Each evening, note:

- Three sensory stressors you experienced
- What helped reduce them
- What you can adjust tomorrow

Patterns will emerge—and with them, your power to create change.

You Deserve to Understand Your Triggers

You're not overreacting. You're responding to inputs your nervous system was never meant to ignore. The fact that others don't notice them doesn't mean they don't affect you.

Identifying your triggers is not about control—it's about compassion. When you understand what overwhelms you, you can make choices that protect your peace, energy, and clarity.

In the next chapter, we'll take this one step further: what can you do *in the moment* when sensory overload hits?

From grounding exercises to emergency exits, you'll learn how to stabilize your system when it feels like it's slipping out of reach.

But for now, just pause.

Breathe.

And remember: recognizing your triggers is the first act of self-respect in a noisy world.

CHAPTER 4: EMERGENCY TOOLS FOR OVERLOAD MOMENTS

What to Do When You're on the Edge of a Shutdown

There comes a moment—whether in the middle of a loud office, a crowded store, or a chaotic family gathering—when everything starts to blur. Your heart races. The sounds feel sharper, the lights brighter, and your thoughts harder to catch. You're not just stressed. You are overloaded.

This is a critical turning point.

In this chapter, we shift from understanding and awareness to **action**. What do you do in the heat of the moment, when the input is too much and you feel like you're about to snap, shut down, or fall apart?

The strategies that follow are not abstract suggestions. They are **emergency tools**—evidence-informed, accessible methods designed to bring your nervous system back to safety when the world feels unsafe.

You don't need to push through. You don't need to override your signals. You need a way back to yourself. And that begins here.

Understanding the Crisis State: Fight, Flight, Freeze

When you're overstimulated, you're likely entering a **sympathetic nervous system response**—commonly known as fight or flight. In some cases, if the overload persists or you feel trapped, your body may move into freeze or shutdown. This is the **parasympathetic dorsal state**, where energy drops, detachment sets in, and everything feels numb or far away.

Both of these responses are biological—not failures. Your system is doing exactly what it was designed to do: protect you. The problem is, in a modern world, these threats are often chronic and subtle. You're not running from a tiger. You're stuck in a meeting, a traffic jam, or a crowded mall—but your brain doesn't know the difference.

The tools in this chapter are designed to **signal safety** to your body. They bring you back into what's known as the **ventral vagal state**—a regulated zone where your system can rest, connect, and think clearly again.

Let's begin with the most accessible techniques.

1. The 5-4-3-2-1 Grounding Technique

This method anchors you to the present by engaging all five senses. It's simple, discreet, and effective for both panic and sensory overload.

How it works:

- Identify **5 things you can see**. Look around and name them.
- Identify **4 things you can touch**. Focus on texture and temperature.
- Identify **3 things you can hear**. Listen deeply.
- Identify **2 things you can smell**. If you can't smell anything, recall a comforting scent.
- Identify **1 thing you can taste**. This can be your breath, a sip of water, or a mint.

Why it helps: It slows your racing mind and reconnects you with the physical world, helping pull you out of spiraling thoughts.

2. Box Breathing (4x4x4x4)

This technique, used by Navy SEALs and therapists alike, is a fast way to regulate breathing and heart rate.

Instructions:

- Inhale for a count of 4
- Hold for a count of 4
- Exhale for a count of 4
- Hold for a count of 4
- Repeat for at least 4 rounds

Why it helps: It activates the vagus nerve, shifting your system away from fight-or-flight into parasympathetic calm.

3. Cold Water Reset

When you're overloaded, your brain needs a physical signal that it's time to stop reacting. Cold exposure provides that interruption.

Options:

- Splash cold water on your face
- Run cold water over your wrists or hands
- Hold a cold compress to your neck or cheeks
- Suck on ice or take a chilled sip of water

Why it helps: Cold activates the mammalian dive reflex, which slows the heart rate and calms the nervous system quickly.

4. Earthing (Ground Contact)

If possible, take off your shoes and stand barefoot on grass, soil, or sand. If you're indoors, try lying on the floor, pressing your palms against a wall, or simply sitting with your feet flat and grounded.

Why it helps: Physical contact with stable surfaces reduces dissociation and reestablishes a sense of safety in the body.

5. Vocal Vibration (Humming or Singing Low Notes)

Stimulating the vagus nerve through sound can create rapid nervous system regulation.

Try this:

- Hum a deep, steady tone
- Sing a comforting song quietly
- Speak low and slowly to yourself ("I'm okay. This will pass.")
- Use a calming app with binaural tones

Why it helps: Sound creates vibrational regulation in your throat and chest, helping shift your body toward calm.

6. Containment: The Safe Place Visualization

When you can't physically leave a situation but need relief, visualization can offer a sensory exit.

Steps:

- Close your eyes (if safe to do so)
- Picture a place where you've felt calm—nature, home, childhood space
- Engage your senses: What do you see, hear, feel, smell, taste?
- Anchor to that space for at least 60 seconds

Why it helps: The brain doesn't fully distinguish between real and imagined stimuli. A calming mental scene can override a chaotic environment.

7. Create a Personal Calm Kit

One of the most effective things you can do is assemble a small, portable toolkit of sensory-regulating items you can carry with you or keep at work.

Calm Kit Essentials:

- Noise-canceling headphones or earplugs
- Sunglasses or blue-light-blocking glasses
- A soft fabric or stim toy

- Essential oils or a scent you find grounding
- A water bottle or mints
- A grounding stone, bead, or fidget ring
- A laminated 5-4-3-2-1 card
- A written self-reminder like "This will pass. You are safe."

Why it helps: Having immediate access to tools reduces panic, provides control, and shortens the duration of overload.

8. The Power of Exit and Recovery

Sometimes, the best tool is permission to leave. Whether it's a room, a conversation, a Zoom call, or an environment, if your nervous system is on the verge of collapse, stepping away is not failure. It's wisdom.

Examples of exit phrases:

- "I need a moment to reset. I'll be back shortly."
- "I need some air—please continue without me."
- "Can we take a short pause?"
- "I'm going to step outside and ground myself."

After the exit, give yourself space. Don't re-engage too soon. Let your body return to baseline.

Build a Ritual, Not a Reaction

These techniques are powerful, but they become even more effective when they're integrated into your life **before** a crisis hits. Start building a personal emergency ritual—a reliable sequence you follow when you feel escalation.

Example Ritual:

1. Step outside or to a private space
2. Splash cold water and take three deep breaths
3. Use 5-4-3-2-1 grounding
4. Apply essential oil or stim with a grounding object
5. Sit quietly and hum for 30 seconds

This creates predictability for your system. Over time, your body will begin to recognize the ritual and respond more quickly.

You're Not Powerless in the Moment

Sensory overload can feel like you've lost control of your mind, your body, or your emotions. But the truth is: you **do** have tools. You **can** influence your state.

The key is to act **before** you hit the breaking point. Learn to recognize early signs:

- Increased heart rate

- Tunnel vision or irritability
- Difficulty hearing or concentrating
- Restlessness or the urge to flee

These are signals. They are invitations—not punishments—to intervene early and care for yourself.

You don't need to endure the entire storm. You can build shelter while it forms.

In the next chapter, we'll explore how to move beyond reactive tools into **long-term lifestyle design**—creating spaces, habits, and schedules that naturally reduce overload and increase resilience.

For now, let this chapter be your pocket-sized lifeline. When the noise gets too loud, when the light becomes too bright, when the moment feels too much—reach for one of these tools.

They're not just techniques.

They're proof that your experience is valid, and your peace is possible.

CHAPTER 5: REDESIGNING YOUR DAILY ENVIRONMENT

Creating Calm Spaces That Support, Not Strain, Your Nervous System

You wake up to a harsh alarm. The overhead light glares the moment you flip the switch. You walk into the kitchen, cluttered with yesterday's dishes and today's decisions. As you scroll through emails under fluorescent lights or try to focus at a noisy desk, you wonder why your shoulders are already tight, your breathing shallow, your brain fog creeping in by 9:00 a.m.

This isn't just stress. This is the **architecture of overwhelm**.

Sensory overload often begins before you've left your house. And unless you consciously design your environment to support your nervous system, you'll spend your days reacting to stimuli instead of moving through them with ease.

The goal of this chapter is simple: help you identify, declutter, and transform the physical and digital spaces where you spend your time—so that they regulate your nervous system, not hijack it.

When your environment becomes an ally instead of an enemy, everything else—focus, calm, productivity, relationships—begins to shift.

Your Environment Is a Nervous System Influencer

The spaces we occupy are not neutral. They interact with our brains and bodies constantly. Every color, sound, texture, and scent is processed by your sensory system, whether you're aware of it or not.

A noisy refrigerator can increase your heart rate. Harsh lighting can trigger a cortisol spike. Clutter can cause the brain to enter a low-grade fight-or-flight response due to perceived chaos and lack of control.

This means the environment you inhabit is **either helping you regulate or contributing to your dysregulation**. The good news? With small, deliberate changes, you can shift the scales dramatically.

Let's begin with the place you start and end your day.

The Bedroom: Reclaiming Rest

Sleep is one of the most powerful tools for sensory resilience. But many people with sensory sensitivity struggle to fall asleep or stay asleep—not due to insomnia alone, but because the environment itself is overstimulating.

Common Triggers:

- Synthetic fabrics that trap heat or feel scratchy
- Bright LED alarm clocks
- Inconsistent lighting from screens or windows
- Background noise from outside traffic or appliances
- Too much visual clutter on nightstands and walls

Supportive Shifts:

- Use blackout curtains to block intrusive light
- Choose natural, breathable fabrics for bedding
- Remove electronics or use airplane mode overnight
- Introduce a weighted blanket if calming pressure is helpful
- Limit bedroom decor to soothing, soft, or earth-toned items
- Keep the space visually minimal and temperature regulated

Your bedroom should feel like a cocoon—not an inbox. Think quiet, warm, and secure. That's where recovery begins.

The Bathroom: Sensory Sanctuary or Source of Stress?

Bathrooms are often overlooked in sensory design, but they can be surprisingly triggering—especially in the morning when you're not yet regulated.

Triggers to Address:

- Bright vanity lighting without dimmer options
- Cold floors or surfaces
- Jarring noise from fans or flushing systems
- Strong chemical smells from cleaners or personal products

Soothing Upgrades:

- Switch to warm white bulbs or install dimmable lighting
- Add a small floor mat or soft slippers for tactile comfort
- Use unscented or naturally scented personal care products
- Keep only daily essentials on counters to reduce visual noise
- Add a plant, calming artwork, or soft textures to balance the space

If your morning routine begins in stress, the rest of your day will struggle to recover. Start with serenity.

The Kitchen: Decision Fatigue and Visual Noise

For many people, the kitchen is both functional and frustrating. It demands rapid decision-making, tolerates clutter, and is often filled with jarring sensory elements like smells, sounds, and temperature shifts.

Common Stressors:

- Overstuffed counters, drawers, and refrigerator doors
- Loud appliances (microwaves, coffee grinders, fans)
- Sharp contrasts in lighting (stove hood vs. room light)
- Overwhelming choices during meal prep

Stabilizing Adjustments:

- Group items by use and reduce visual clutter
- Store items in opaque bins or drawers to calm the visual field
- Add soft, under-cabinet lighting for early morning or evening use
- Use earplugs during loud appliance use if needed

- Prep meals in advance to minimize peak-time decision pressure

A well-ordered kitchen restores not just the stomach, but the mind.

The Living Room or Workspace: Where Your Brain Works or Shuts Down

Whether you're remote working, caregiving, freelancing, or relaxing—your primary daytime environment impacts your mental clarity and mood more than you might realize.

Hidden Agitators:

- Open-plan layouts with multiple visual inputs
- Background noise from TV, street traffic, or neighbors
- Too many screens, open tabs, or alerts
- Poor seating ergonomics that create physical tension

Nervous-System-Friendly Shifts:

- Anchor your space with one calming focal point (plant, artwork, or candle)
- Use noise-canceling headphones, white noise, or calming playlists

- Turn off visual notifications and create screen boundaries
- Position your workspace near natural light if possible
- Keep only essential items in your field of vision
- Declutter regularly and maintain a "reset zone" you return to daily

Your environment is an extension of your inner world. Create visual simplicity, and your mind will follow.

Clothing as Micro-Environment

While not a room in your home, your clothing functions as your **portable environment**. It travels with you into every sensory encounter.

Tactile Triggers:

- Tight waistbands or seams
- Itchy tags or fabrics
- Clothes that retain heat or feel stiff
- Outfits that require constant adjustment

Supportive Clothing Tips:

- Choose softness, stretch, and breathability over style trends

- Remove tags, avoid synthetics if they irritate
- Have go-to "calm clothes" for regulation days
- Invest in textures and fits that feel good, not just look good

Your comfort is not a vanity—it's a safety signal.

The Digital Environment: Invisible, Yet Loud

Even the most tranquil physical space can be shattered by an overstimulating digital one. Your phone, inbox, browser, and apps form a **digital landscape** that can feel just as overwhelming as a cluttered room.

Digital Disruptors:

- Constant pings, vibrations, or pop-up notifications
- Social media scroll loops
- Email inbox overload
- Visual clutter from too many open tabs or programs

Digital Design Strategies:

- Use "Do Not Disturb" or focus modes throughout the day
- Turn off nonessential notifications
- Unsubscribe from unused mailing lists

- Use calming wallpaper and reduce screen brightness
- Batch-check emails and social media, don't let them drip-feed stimulation
- Use noise-friendly fonts and soft color schemes if reading for long periods

Minimalism in your digital space restores your attention and decreases micro-stressors.

Sensory Buffer Zones

If redesigning every space feels too ambitious, start with a **single buffer zone**—a small corner, chair, or room designed entirely for decompression. No devices. No obligations. Just presence and peace.

Ideas for a Buffer Zone:

- A cozy chair with a blanket, soft lighting, and calming scents
- A small corner with headphones, stim objects, or reading material
- A closet-turned-calm-nook with textures you enjoy
- A standing mat and journal next to your bed for sensory check-ins

This doesn't have to be elaborate. It just needs to be consistent, accessible, and regulated.

Transformation Is in the Details

When your environment is in harmony with your nervous system, something extraordinary happens. You stop bracing. You stop flinching. You stop enduring. You start living.

Every drawer you declutter, every light you soften, every texture you choose with care—these are not aesthetic upgrades. They are **acts of self-respect**.

Don't underestimate the power of micro-adjustments. They build into macro-changes. As your surroundings begin to soothe you, your internal state will follow.

In the next chapter, we'll explore the next layer of support—**boundaries**. Not just physical ones, but emotional and social ones that protect your sensory energy and help you advocate for your needs without shame.

For now, look around your space. Choose one change to make today. One corner. One drawer. One lightbulb.

And let that change begin to speak safety to your body.

CHAPTER 6: SETTING BOUNDARIES WITHOUT GUILT

How to Communicate Your Needs Without Apologizing for Them

For many adults who live with sensory sensitivity, the hardest part isn't identifying what overwhelms them. It's protecting themselves from it—especially when that means saying no to other people.

Boundaries are difficult for anyone who has been socialized to prioritize harmony, performance, or approval. For those with sensory needs, boundary-setting becomes even more complex. You may feel like you're the only one asking for silence in a loud room. Or like you're the one who always leaves the party early, avoids group chats, or declines invitations at the last minute.

You might wonder: Will they think I'm rude? Inflexible? Difficult? Will I be seen as antisocial or weak?

This chapter is not just about learning to say no. It's about learning to say yes—to your limits, your body, your right to exist in a world that isn't built with your nervous system in mind.

We will explore how to set boundaries that preserve your energy, reduce guilt, and foster mutual understanding in both personal and professional relationships.

Because when your boundaries are clear, your relationships become clearer too.

The Emotional Weight of Saying No

Let's start by acknowledging something most guides skip over: saying no can feel painful. Especially if you've been raised in an environment where compliance, performance, or emotional labor was rewarded.

Many adults with sensory sensitivity also score high in empathy. You feel what others feel. You don't want to disappoint or inconvenience anyone. And so, you say yes—even when your body says no.

But over time, this creates emotional and physiological debt. Every time you override your needs, your body pays the price.

The goal here is not to become rigid or controlling. The goal is to become **self-respecting**. And that begins with recognizing that your energy is not infinite, your presence is not obligatory, and your regulation is not optional—it's essential.

What Are Sensory Boundaries?

Sensory boundaries are the limits you set to protect your nervous system from overstimulation. These boundaries are not arbitrary—they are based on direct, lived experience of what helps you function and what causes you to shut down.

Sensory boundaries may include:

- Limiting time in noisy or crowded environments
- Saying no to back-to-back meetings or social events
- Requesting lower lighting or quiet spaces when possible
- Wearing headphones or sunglasses in overstimulating places
- Turning off phone notifications during recovery time
- Asking others not to touch you unexpectedly
- Leaving events early without needing to justify

These are not signs of avoidance or fragility. They are **adaptive strategies**. Just as someone with a food allergy avoids certain ingredients, someone with a sensitive nervous system avoids environments that trigger distress.

How to Recognize When You Need a Boundary

You may not always know in advance when something will overwhelm you. But over time, your body develops patterns. Learning to recognize your early signs of overload is essential.

Here are some indicators that you need a boundary:

- You feel pressure in your chest or tightness in your jaw
- You notice irritability, even with people you care about
- You begin dreading events you normally enjoy
- You experience decision fatigue or can't think clearly
- You feel resentment toward others for "asking too much"
- You fantasize about disappearing or canceling everything

These signals are not overreactions. They are *invitations*— clear prompts from your nervous system asking you to draw a line, take space, or protect your energy.

Boundaries are not walls. They are filters. They let in what supports you and screen out what drains you.

Boundary Scripts: What to Say and How to Say It

One of the most effective ways to reduce guilt around boundaries is to prepare your language in advance. When you know what to say, you're less likely to freeze or apologize.

Here are scripts tailored to common scenarios:

Workplace Boundaries

- "I work best in quiet environments. Would it be possible to book a room or use headphones during our collaborative sessions?"
- "I'll need time between meetings to regroup. Can we space them out or add buffer time?"
- "I'm happy to contribute, but I'll need to step out after 45 minutes. That's my current limit for focus and noise."
- "For sensory reasons, I don't attend video calls with multiple screens on. I'll join by voice if that works."

Social Boundaries

- "Thanks so much for the invite. I'm limiting my evening plans this week to recharge, but I hope to connect soon."

- "Large group settings can be tough on my system. Can we do something more low-key or one-on-one?"
- "I may need to leave early depending on how I'm feeling, but I'd love to stop by for a while."
- "I'm not ignoring you—I'm in a sensory recovery window. I'll respond when I've reset."

Family and Home Boundaries

- "I need a quiet space for an hour to regulate. I'll be back after that."
- "Let's plan visits during times when I'm more grounded—late evenings are difficult for me."
- "Please avoid loud sounds when possible. I know it's not always easy, but it helps me stay present."
- "I love spending time with you, and I also need breaks to rest my system. Both are true."

Notice the pattern in these scripts. They:

- State the need clearly
- Take ownership without blame
- Offer alternative options when possible
- Reflect care for both parties
- Do not over-explain or apologize

You're not asking for special treatment. You're asking for alignment with how your brain and body function best.

The Guilt Myth: You're Not Letting Anyone Down

One of the biggest blocks to boundary-setting is guilt. You worry you're disappointing others, damaging relationships, or being "difficult."

But guilt is not always a reliable emotion. Sometimes, guilt is a sign that you're breaking a pattern of self-abandonment—not that you're doing something wrong.

Ask yourself:

- Am I feeling guilty because I hurt someone?
- Or because I said yes to myself for the first time in a long time?

You can care deeply about others and still choose yourself. In fact, people in your life benefit more when you are **regulated, present, and emotionally available**—not exhausted, overstimulated, or resentful.

Boundaries are not punishments. They are investments in long-term connection.

What If People Don't Understand?

Not everyone will understand your sensory needs right away. Some may question them. Some may push back. Others may interpret your boundaries as rejection.

This is painful—but it is not a reason to abandon yourself.

You can explain your needs with grace, but you cannot control how others respond. And if someone repeatedly dismisses, mocks, or violates your boundaries, it may be time to reevaluate the role they play in your life.

The people who belong in your circle are the ones who *make room* for your regulation, not just your participation.

Micro-Boundaries: Small Acts of Self-Protection

Not all boundaries require formal conversations. You can also use **micro-boundaries**—subtle shifts that protect your energy without requiring explanation.

Examples include:

- Lowering the volume or brightness on your devices
- Driving alone instead of carpooling
- Using noise-canceling earbuds at home

- Turning off your phone during sensory recovery hours
- Wearing sunglasses or hats in bright spaces
- Pre-scheduling "do not disturb" blocks into your calendar

These changes may seem small, but they signal something powerful: that your regulation matters. That your nervous system is not something to be ignored. That you are worthy of a life designed to support, not suppress, your needs.

Boundaries Are Not Barriers. They Are Bridges.

When you begin setting boundaries, your relationships may shift. Some will deepen. Some will fade. Some may surprise you with grace and understanding.

The most important relationship that will change is the one with yourself.

You will begin to feel safer in your own body. More grounded in your choices. Less reactive, and more at peace.

Boundaries are not the end of connection. They are the beginning of **true connection**—based not on performance or endurance, but on mutual care and respect.

In the next chapter, we move from interpersonal boundaries to internal restoration. You'll learn how to listen to your body more deeply—through rest, movement, nutrition, and sensory-friendly routines that nourish your system from the inside out.

But before we go there, take a moment now.

Name one area where your body is asking for a boundary.

And consider this: what would it feel like to say yes to that request?

You are allowed to protect your peace.

You are allowed to be well.

And the people who truly see you will never need you to suffer to stay close.

CHAPTER 7: WHEN SENSORY OVERLOAD IMPACTS MENTAL HEALTH

Understanding the Link Between Overstimulation, Anxiety, and Emotional Exhaustion

There comes a point when it's no longer just about the noise or the lights or the clutter. It's not just that you're sensitive to sounds or that crowds drain you. It's something deeper, heavier, and harder to shake.

You begin to feel tired all the time. But not just tired— empty. You forget small things. You cry unexpectedly. You lose patience quickly. You dread leaving the house or opening your inbox. And you can't remember the last time your body felt truly calm.

Sensory overload, when persistent and unmanaged, doesn't stay confined to your environment. Over time, it starts to impact your **mental health**, your sense of identity, and your emotional well-being.

This chapter is about understanding that impact—and learning how to begin reversing it.

You are not broken. But you may be carrying more input, tension, and unresolved stress than your nervous system was designed to handle.

And you're not alone.

Chronic Overload Is More Than a Sensory Issue

When we think of sensory overload, we often imagine momentary episodes—a loud room, a flashing light, an irritating fabric. But for many adults, especially those without supportive systems, the overload is **ongoing**. It becomes a **background condition**, not a one-time event.

Living in a state of near-constant overstimulation can lead to symptoms that are commonly misdiagnosed as purely psychological:

- Chronic anxiety or panic attacks
- Emotional volatility or numbness
- Depression or low mood
- Burnout and mental fatigue
- Social withdrawal
- Hypervigilance
- Loss of motivation or concentration
- Irritability that feels disproportionate
- Trouble sleeping or relaxing

These are not signs of personal failure. They are signs of **nervous system exhaustion**.

When your body is constantly on high alert, the boundary between sensory and emotional becomes blurred. You may think you're emotionally unstable, when in reality, your nervous system is overworked, under-supported, and never allowed to fully reset.

The Overlap Between Sensory Sensitivity and Anxiety

Anxiety is often the first mental health diagnosis received by adults with sensory overload. That's because the symptoms overlap so closely.

Anxiety, at its core, is the body's alarm system going off too frequently or too intensely. Sensory overload can trigger that same alarm—sometimes repeatedly, in ways that feel uncontrollable or irrational.

For example:

- A noisy café feels unsafe, even though nothing "bad" is happening
- A crowded bus ride causes nausea and chest tightness
- A simple phone call induces dread and panic

- A full inbox sparks shame and spiraling thoughts

These aren't overreactions. They're your nervous system trying to interpret a high volume of input and assigning urgency to what it doesn't have capacity to sort through.

You're not imagining the tension. You're experiencing it— deeply, viscerally, and chronically.

Burnout: The Final Stage of Constant Overload

Burnout isn't just for high-achieving professionals or overworked parents. Burnout is what happens when **your internal resources are depleted faster than they are replenished**, over and over again.

For sensory-sensitive adults, burnout can look like:

- Emotional detachment or feeling "checked out"
- Cynicism, irritability, or hopelessness
- Losing interest in things you used to enjoy
- Feeling like you're just "going through the motions"
- Resisting social contact, even with people you love
- A desire to disappear, not because of depression, but because of sheer exhaustion

This is not laziness. This is not apathy. This is **survival mode**, prolonged past its safe limits.

Your body has been sounding the alarm for too long without relief. Eventually, it shuts down to protect you.

Recognizing burnout is the first step toward recovery. And the good news is: your body wants to heal. It just needs time, safety, and nourishment to do so.

Emotional Dysregulation and Shutdown

Another common mental health effect of sensory overload is **emotional dysregulation**—an inability to manage or understand your emotional responses.

This can mean:

- Crying easily and unpredictably
- Feeling like your reactions are too big for the situation
- Experiencing anger or fear that feels unprovoked
- Going numb or feeling nothing at all
- Struggling to articulate how you feel

Emotional dysregulation isn't just about trauma or mood disorders. It's often a direct consequence of living in environments that repeatedly overwhelm your sensory system without giving you time or tools to recover.

When your body is overstimulated, it loses the energy and clarity required to process emotions effectively. You may not be emotionally volatile—you may simply be emotionally **overloaded**.

And when you don't have language for what you're feeling, your relationships, self-esteem, and confidence begin to suffer.

This is not a character flaw. This is a **signal** that your nervous system is carrying more than it can hold.

The Psychology of Shame and Isolation

One of the most painful outcomes of unmanaged sensory overload is **shame**.

Shame tells you:

- "Other people can handle this. Why can't you?"
- "You're just being dramatic."
- "You're a burden to your friends or coworkers."
- "You're too sensitive for real life."
- "No one will understand you."

Shame leads to silence. Silence leads to isolation. And isolation leads to worsening symptoms, because without validation or language, your experiences remain internalized.

But here's the truth:

You are not weak. You are not broken. You are living in a world that moves at a volume, speed, and intensity that your nervous system cannot sustainably match. That doesn't make you less capable. It makes you **different**— and worthy of different care.

You may not need medication. You may not need endless therapy sessions. You may simply need **a life with fewer triggers and more space**. A life that respects your internal pace. A life where emotional equilibrium is possible again.

How to Begin Healing the Mind-Body System

Recovery from sensory-related emotional distress isn't instant. It is a process of re-patterning your days, your decisions, and your environments to offer your system **what it has long been denied**—relief, respect, and regulation.

Here's where you can begin.

1. Prioritize Emotional Safety Over Performance

Give yourself permission to under-function while you recover. Cancel plans. Decline invitations. Choose stillness over stimulation, even if it feels selfish. Your nervous system will not heal in a state of constant demand.

2. Practice Name-It-to-Tame-It

Use simple language to describe what you're feeling. "I feel flooded." "I feel disconnected." "I feel overstimulated." Naming your internal state reduces shame and gives your brain a sense of control.

3. Create Emotional Check-In Points

Schedule pauses in your day to assess how you feel. Ask: Am I grounded? Am I overwhelmed? Do I need a reset? This creates self-trust and early intervention before escalation occurs.

4. Reduce All Non-Essential Inputs

Give your system space by cutting back on noise, notifications, screen time, and multitasking. Every reduction frees up capacity for regulation and recovery.

5. Journal Without Pressure

Write one paragraph per day describing your internal weather. Use sensory terms: "foggy," "buzzing," "cold," "static," "shaky." This builds emotional literacy and helps you track patterns.

6. Seek Regulating Relationships

Spend time with people who are calm, slow-paced, and validating. Even brief exposure to these relational dynamics can begin to recalibrate your internal rhythms.

7. Integrate Somatic Practices

Try gentle yoga, slow walking, stretching, rocking, or touch-based regulation. These practices reconnect the body and brain, easing shutdown and panic through physical reassurance.

You Are Not Your Dysregulation

It can be difficult to separate yourself from your symptoms. But who you are is not defined by your anxiety, burnout, or shutdowns. These are **responses**, not identities.

They are your body's attempt to stay safe in an unsafe environment. They are evidence of your survival, not your brokenness.

As you move through the rest of this book, you'll gather tools for redesigning your routines, your relationships, and your rest—not to eliminate sensitivity, but to finally support it.

In the next chapter, we turn toward **nourishment**. Because your nervous system isn't just influenced by sound or light—it's shaped by what you eat, how you sleep, and the rhythms you build into your body. You'll learn how to partner with your physiology, not fight it, and begin building a lifestyle that heals from the inside out.

But before we move on, take a moment to tell yourself something you may not have heard in a long time:

It makes sense that you feel this way.
You are allowed to feel this way.
And you do not have to stay this way.

There is a way forward.

And it begins with honoring the truth of what you feel.

CHAPTER 8: NOURISH THE BODY, CALM THE SENSES

Supporting Your Nervous System Through Food, Sleep, Hydration, and Movement

Your nervous system does not exist in isolation. It is not a floating mechanism reacting to lights and sounds in a vacuum. It is embedded in a **body**—a living, breathing, sensing organism that requires fuel, rest, and rhythm to function well.

When your body is depleted, your sensory resilience drops. You become more reactive to sound, more sensitive to light, more easily overwhelmed by texture, touch, or smell. This is not just psychological. It is **physiological**.

And it is often overlooked.

In this chapter, we explore the **foundational pillars** of nervous system regulation that begin in the body: what you eat, how you sleep, how you hydrate, and how you move.

These may sound basic. But they are the ground floor of all other healing. Without nourishment, no amount of strategy will stick. Without rest, no boundaries will hold. Without hydration or gentle movement, your regulation will remain fragile.

This chapter is about building strength—not through willpower or intensity, but through softness, slowness, and consistency.

Because sensory wellness begins in the body long before it shows up in the mind.

Food as Regulation, Not Reward or Restriction

Many adults eat based on convenience, shame, emotional coping, or habit. Few eat with their **nervous system** in mind.

But food is not just about calories. It is information. It tells your body whether to activate or calm. To fight or to restore.

Certain nutrients are especially supportive for sensory-sensitive individuals because they impact neurotransmitters, inflammation, and stress hormones.

Key Nutritional Foundations for Sensory Wellness:

1. **Magnesium-Rich Foods**
   Magnesium helps regulate the stress response system. It supports muscle relaxation, reduces irritability, and calms the central nervous system.

   Sources: Leafy greens, almonds, cashews, black beans, pumpkin seeds, avocado, dark chocolate (in moderation)

2. **Omega-3 Fatty Acids**
   Omega-3s reduce neuroinflammation and improve brain resilience, which can lower sensory reactivity and support mood regulation.

   Sources: Fatty fish (salmon, mackerel), walnuts, chia seeds, flaxseed, seaweed

3. **Complex Carbohydrates**
   Carbs support serotonin production, which contributes to emotional stability and calm. Choose complex carbs that release energy slowly.

   Sources: Brown rice, oats, lentils, sweet potatoes, quinoa

4. **Hydrating, Whole Foods**
   Many people are under-hydrated from processed

food. Fresh fruits and vegetables offer water, fiber, and micronutrients all at once.

Sources: Cucumber, celery, watermelon, oranges, strawberries, leafy greens

5. **Protein for Stabilization**
   Protein supports dopamine and serotonin synthesis and helps maintain blood sugar levels, which influence mood and focus.

   Sources: Eggs, legumes, tofu, poultry, nuts, seeds, dairy, beans

Avoiding Extreme Dieting:
Sensory overload becomes worse when blood sugar drops, digestion is poor, or the body lacks basic fuel. Avoid restrictive eating plans unless medically necessary. Your nervous system needs **stability**, not volatility.

Eat regularly. Choose whole foods. Listen to how different meals affect your clarity and calm.

This is not about perfection. It's about partnership—with your body, not against it.

Hydration: The Forgotten Regulator

Mild dehydration can mimic or exacerbate symptoms of anxiety, fatigue, brain fog, and overwhelm. Many adults with sensory overload are chronically under-hydrated—not by choice, but by distraction, disconnection, or dysregulation.

What Proper Hydration Does:

- Improves cognitive processing
- Supports thermoregulation (reducing heat-related sensory distress)
- Eases irritability and low mood
- Helps with digestion, reducing internal discomfort
- Enhances energy and emotional regulation

Tips for Gentle Hydration:

- Begin your morning with a glass of water before caffeine
- Add a slice of lemon, cucumber, or mint for sensory interest
- Use a water bottle with a soft straw or spout if textures help
- Track your intake without obsessing—aim for consistent sipping over the day

Don't wait until you're thirsty. Thirst is a late-stage signal. Create a routine where water is woven into your environment.

It may seem small. But hydration is one of the fastest ways to return to internal balance.

Sleep: Where Restoration Begins

Sensory overload and sleep disturbance often go hand in hand. You may struggle to fall asleep because your nervous system remains alert. Or you may wake up frequently, your body still on high alert even in rest.

This cycle becomes self-reinforcing. Poor sleep leads to lower tolerance the next day. Overload then leads to another restless night.

Sleep is not just rest. It is **repair**. During deep sleep, the brain clears out toxins, downregulates stress hormones, and resets sensory filters.

Sleep Support for Sensitive Adults:

1. **Dim lights two hours before bedtime** to signal melatonin production
2. **Avoid stimulating content or social media at night**—your brain will remain engaged

3. **Create a wind-down ritual:** light stretching, tea, calming music, scent cues like lavender
4. **Use white noise or gentle soundscapes** to buffer environmental disruptions
5. **Keep your bedroom cool, dark, and tech-free** when possible
6. **Go to bed and wake up at the same time each day**, even on weekends
7. **Use weighted blankets or soft textures** if tactile input soothes you

If falling asleep is a struggle, focus first on consistency. Sleep hygiene is not a quick fix, but a practice. And it is one of the most powerful tools you have.

Movement: Not Fitness—Regulation

Many sensory-sensitive adults struggle with exercise, either because traditional workouts feel overwhelming or because gym environments are too stimulating.

But **movement is medicine**—when done mindfully. You don't need a rigorous routine. You need **rhythm**.

Movement supports sensory wellness by:

- Releasing built-up tension
- Supporting lymphatic drainage and detox

- Boosting mood through endorphin release
- Improving sleep quality
- Enhancing proprioception (awareness of body in space)
- Resetting the stress response through breath and repetition

Nervous-System-Friendly Movement Ideas:

- Walking in nature or quiet areas
- Gentle stretching or slow yoga
- Dancing alone to calming music
- Tai chi, qigong, or water-based movement
- Rocking in a chair or gentle self-swaying
- Foam rolling or soft tissue release
- Breath-linked movement (inhale, reach; exhale, release)

Avoid competitive, overstimulating fitness environments if they worsen your symptoms. You're not lazy if you don't go to a gym. You're wise to move in ways that nourish rather than drain.

The goal is not to sculpt or sweat. The goal is to come back into your body—to feel it as **yours**, not as something constantly reacting to the world.

Food, hydration, sleep, and movement are not isolated tasks. They work in tandem to create a rhythm—a **sensory-supportive cadence** that gives your body the signal: you are safe now.

If you've lived for years in a state of depletion or anxiety, these basics may feel insignificant at first. They are not. They are the soil from which regulation grows.

Start small.

- Add one magnesium-rich food to your meals
- Keep a water bottle on your desk or bedside
- Stretch your arms overhead each morning
- Turn off your screens 30 minutes earlier
- Walk for five minutes without a podcast or task

Let these be acts of nourishment, not discipline. Restoration, not repair.

Your body is not your enemy. It is your **first ally** in calming the world inside and outside of you.

You Deserve to Be Well-Fed, Well-Rested, and Well-Cared For

If you were never taught to care for your body gently, this may feel foreign. If you've internalized a push-through mentality, slowing down may trigger guilt. If you've lived in environments where sensitivity was dismissed, prioritizing your wellness may feel selfish.

But your health—mental, sensory, emotional—is not a luxury. It is the foundation upon which everything else rests.

You are allowed to eat slowly. To sleep deeply. To move gently. To hydrate intentionally. These are not indulgences. They are acts of radical alignment with your nature.

In the next chapter, we expand outward again—into the realm of relationships. How can sensory-sensitive adults navigate connection, intimacy, and belonging while honoring their limits? How can partners, friends, and loved ones learn to support without overstepping?

But before we go there, return to your body now. Ask it what it needs.

Not what it *should* need.

What it *actually* needs.

And begin there.

CHAPTER 9: LOVE, FRIENDSHIP, AND SENSORY DIFFERENCES

Navigating Relationships While Honoring Your Nervous System

For many sensory-sensitive adults, relationships are both a source of comfort and a source of stress. You long for connection—deep, meaningful, emotionally safe connection—but you may find that the very things others expect in relationships can overwhelm you.

You may love someone deeply and still find their presence exhausting after too long. You may enjoy socializing in theory, but dread the reality of noise, unpredictability, and overstimulation. You may feel closest to people who respect your space, yet worry that asking for too much space might alienate them.

Relationships for sensory-sensitive people are not impossible. But they do require honesty, structure, and communication that is often missing from traditional relationship advice.

This chapter will help you build and sustain healthy connections—romantic, platonic, familial—while staying true to your own needs. You don't have to choose between love and peace. You deserve both.

The Sensory Landscape of Connection

Let's start by naming what's often unspoken: intimacy, friendship, and closeness all come with **sensory expectations**. Hugs, conversations, shared meals, sleepovers, public gatherings, phone calls, physical affection—these are baked into most relationships without question.

But for someone with a sensitive nervous system, each of these things may carry **hidden costs**.

- Physical affection may feel overwhelming, even from someone you love
- Shared spaces may bring sensory overload from lighting, sound, or smell
- Phone calls may drain more energy than texts
- Group hangouts may feel chaotic or unmanageable
- Unstructured time together may create anxiety around not being able to withdraw

These are not signs that you're cold, distant, or emotionally unavailable. They are signs that your system is processing relational input differently than others. You care deeply. But your care requires **space**, not just proximity.

When your boundaries are misunderstood or unspoken, relationships can become filled with guilt, resentment, or silence. But when you express your needs clearly, with compassion and conviction, something transformative happens:

Connection begins to feel safe again.

Why Sensory Needs Are Often Misread

Sensory-sensitive people are often mischaracterized in relationships. Common misinterpretations include:

- Needing alone time = being avoidant or disinterested
- Avoiding group events = being antisocial
- Needing to leave early = being dramatic or high-maintenance
- Disliking hugs = being cold or unaffectionate
- Struggling with communication = being passive-aggressive
- Being quiet or observant = being judgmental

These misunderstandings can erode trust on both sides.

You start to internalize shame. You begin to perform connection rather than experience it. You force yourself to endure what your nervous system cannot handle—and then wonder why you feel exhausted, withdrawn, or disconnected afterward.

This dynamic is not sustainable.

Relationships that support your well-being must be **built on clarity**, not compliance. That means educating the people in your life about how your nervous system works— not as an excuse, but as a framework for mutual understanding.

How to Communicate Your Sensory Needs Without Apology

Healthy communication around sensory differences begins with **owning your experience** without self-judgment.

Here are a few examples of how to explain your needs in ways that feel confident and clear:

- "I love spending time with you, and I also need regular quiet time to reset. It's not personal—it's part of how I stay grounded."
- "I feel most present in one-on-one settings. Group events can be overstimulating, so I may decline sometimes even though I care."

- "When I feel overwhelmed, I may go quiet or take space. That's how I regulate—it doesn't mean I'm upset or withdrawing from you emotionally."
- "I love physical closeness, but I may need breaks or non-touch affection depending on how my system is doing."
- "Let's plan something with an exit option. Knowing I can leave when needed helps me stay calmer and more connected while I'm there."

These kinds of statements do several things at once:

- Normalize your sensory experience
- Create context for your behavior
- Affirm care and respect for the relationship
- Offer solutions instead of ultimatums

You don't need to over-explain. You don't need to convince. You just need to speak your truth consistently enough that it becomes a **shared language**.

Designing Sensory-Friendly Relationships

Every relationship is a dynamic between two nervous systems. When your nervous system is more sensitive, it may require more intentional structuring than others are used to. That doesn't make you difficult. It makes you a **conscious partner or friend**.

Here are some ideas for creating relationships that support rather than strain you:

1. Establish Rituals of Connection, Not Obligation
Set up predictable ways to connect that don't rely on spontaneity or overstimulation. A quiet dinner at home. A weekly check-in walk. A Sunday text ritual. Structure provides safety.

2. Use Signals Instead of Explanations
When words are hard in the moment, use pre-agreed signals. A squeeze of the hand that means "I need to step away." A text that means "overloaded, but thinking of you." Non-verbal tools reduce friction and misunderstanding.

3. Offer Alternatives, Not Just Declines
If you say no to a plan, offer another way to connect. "That gathering feels like too much for me, but I'd love to have coffee with you one-on-one this week." This keeps the connection alive while protecting your limits.

4. Plan Recovery Time Around Social Events
Don't stack multiple events or obligations. Create buffer zones. Let your friends and partner know that your absence isn't distance—it's maintenance. You're refueling so you can keep showing up.

5. Share Resources or Articles

Sometimes the people in your life don't understand because they've never been exposed to these concepts. Share a chapter. Share a podcast. Share this book. Education fosters empathy.

6. Acknowledge Their Experience Too

Sensory accommodations go both ways. If a partner or friend is extroverted or highly physical, validate their needs too. "I know it's hard when I need more space. I really appreciate your patience."

Mutual understanding doesn't mean you become someone you're not. It means you build bridges from who you both are—and walk them together.

Intimacy and Sensory Regulation

For many adults, romantic or sexual relationships bring additional layers of sensory complexity. Physical closeness, shared spaces, unpredictable body rhythms—these can all trigger overwhelm, even in loving partnerships.

Here's what helps:

- **Talk about touch**: Discuss what feels grounding versus overwhelming. Where, when, and how affection is offered matters.

- **Plan connection**: Spontaneity isn't a requirement for intimacy. Scheduled time can be just as meaningful, and more comfortable.
- **Sleep separately if needed**: Sensory-sensitive adults often sleep better alone. Normalize this as a care strategy, not rejection.
- **Build quiet connection**: Not all intimacy is physical. Reading together, breathing in sync, silent walks—these are deep forms of bonding too.

Intimacy thrives not from intensity, but from attunement. The more your partner understands your sensory world, the safer your body will feel in theirs.

Grief, Growth, and Letting Go

Sometimes, despite your best efforts, not every relationship will survive the honesty of your sensory boundaries. People may pull away. You may outgrow dynamics based on masking or performance. You may realize that a friendship built on constant compromise no longer fits the person you are becoming.

This is painful—but not tragic.

Letting go is not failure. It is the cost of alignment. And as you make space, you will attract relationships that feel peaceful, mutual, and regulating.

You will begin to feel **chosen** not for your endurance, but for your presence.

You will be loved in your quietness, your slowness, your rhythms.

And those are the connections that last.

The People Who See You Will Stay

You do not have to choose between being yourself and being loved.

The people who are meant to walk beside you will not resent your boundaries. They will admire your self-awareness. They will adjust with you, not around you. They will learn your nervous system the way people learn a language—slowly, imperfectly, but with care.

And you will offer the same in return.

In the final chapter, we move into reflection and empowerment. You've now learned how to understand, manage, and live with sensory overload. But what does it mean to thrive—not just survive—with a sensitive nervous system in a noisy world?

Before we go there, take a moment to honor yourself.

You are building something rare. Relationships rooted in clarity, care, and capacity.

And those are the kinds of love that hold.

EPILOGUE: YOU'RE NOT BROKEN—YOU'RE BUILT DIFFERENTLY

A Closing Reflection for the Sensory-Sensitive Adult

Some books are meant to teach. Some are meant to soothe. This one was always meant to do both.

If you've made it here, through every chapter of reflection, action, and insight, then you've done more than read a book. You've engaged in a deep act of reclamation—the process of returning to yourself after years of disconnection, misunderstanding, and quiet survival.

There is no diagnosis in these pages. No label to define you. Instead, there is permission—permission to feel what you feel, to want what you want, and to care for your nervous system in a way that doesn't wait for crisis.

Let's name the truth clearly, one final time:

You are not too much. You are not too fragile. You are not broken.

You are built differently.

And once you understand that, everything begins to change.

You've Been Living on the Edge of Overload

Perhaps for years.

You've been enduring environments not designed for your sensory wiring. You've been navigating relationships without the language to express what drains or nourishes you. You've been masking your discomfort in order to function, to belong, to be enough.

This comes with a cost. And you've paid it—often in silence.

You've blamed yourself for irritability, brain fog, or the need to withdraw. You've felt guilt for avoiding calls, skipping parties, or leaving early. You've questioned your capacity to cope when others seem unfazed.

But what others can tolerate is not the measure of your strength.

Your sensitivity is not a flaw to fix. It is a **capacity** to honor.

The goal has never been to toughen you up. The goal is to **make the world softer where it can be softened—** and to strengthen your self-understanding where it cannot.

This is how you protect your peace without losing your power.

The Journey You've Taken

Across these chapters, you've learned to see the full shape of your sensory experience. You've named your triggers, recognized the signs of overload, and gathered tools to intervene with grace.

You've learned how to:

- Identify what overwhelms you and why
- Ground yourself in moments of rising tension
- Redesign your home and workspaces for calm
- Nourish your body with food, water, sleep, and movement
- Set clear boundaries without apology
- Communicate your needs in relationships
- Recognize when mental health struggles are rooted in sensory depletion
- Reclaim rest as a right, not a reward

These are not small steps. They are foundational shifts.

And while this book may be ending, the journey of self-regulation and self-respect continues. Not as a finish line to cross, but as a **practice**—daily, gentle, imperfect, and resilient.

You Are Now the Expert on Your Own Nervous System

That may not have always been true. You may have been told what to feel, how to act, what to tolerate. You may have followed others' rhythms at the expense of your own.

But now you know.

You know what overwhelm feels like before it explodes.
You know how to return to calm when your system spikes.
You know how to shape your environment instead of enduring it.
You know what to say when someone doesn't understand.
You know the difference between rest and avoidance.
You know the cost of silence. And the power of voice.

That knowledge cannot be taken from you. It is lived. It is earned. It is yours.

And with it, you can begin building a life that doesn't just accommodate your sensitivity—but is actually shaped by it.

What Thriving Might Look Like for You

Thriving with a sensitive nervous system doesn't look like boundless energy or constant productivity. It doesn't mean you never get overwhelmed again. It doesn't mean you stop needing space, rest, or quiet.

It looks like **living in sync** with yourself.

It looks like choosing slower mornings because that's when you feel centered.
It looks like creating a home that feels like a sanctuary, not a holding cell.
It looks like saying no with kindness and without guilt.
It looks like surrounding yourself with people who don't need you to shrink.
It looks like knowing when to leave, and when to lean in.
It looks like understanding the difference between stimulation and connection.
It looks like planning your week around your energy, not your obligations.
It looks like creating a world where your nervous system is safe enough to let you be fully present, fully human, and fully at peace.

And you don't have to get there all at once. Small steps, taken consistently, build lives that feel sustainable. And that is the true definition of thriving.

Your Sensitivity Is a Strength

Let's go even further.

Your sensitivity is not just something to manage. It's a **strength**—when properly supported.

It allows you to:

- Notice details others miss
- Sense emotional shifts with accuracy
- Anticipate needs before they're voiced
- Create environments that feel deeply nurturing
- Offer empathy with precision
- Protect your peace with discernment
- Experience joy, beauty, and meaning in intense, textured ways

The world needs this.

But the world needs it **from people who are well**.

Not overextended. Not constantly triggered. Not forced into exhaustion to keep up.

That's why your boundaries matter. That's why your lifestyle design matters. That's why your regulation matters.

Because the healthier you are, the more clearly your gifts can emerge.

Sensitivity without support becomes survival.

Sensitivity with support becomes **wisdom**.

Final Words as You Continue Forward

There will be days when it's hard. You will forget tools. You will override your signals. You will feel pulled back into old rhythms.

That's okay.

This is not about perfection. This is about building a relationship with yourself that you never learned to have.

So on those days, return to the basics:

Slow your breath.
Drink water.
Step outside.
Turn off the noise.
Name how you feel.
Say no if needed.
Rest if possible.
Begin again.

You will not always need a crisis to justify your care. You can start now. Without proof. Without collapse.

Just because you are worthy of it.

You were not meant to live in a world that overwhelms you every day. But you were meant to **create space within it**—a space where you feel calm, seen, and whole.

Let that space begin inside of you.

And let it expand—one boundary, one breath, one quiet morning at a time.

You are not broken.

You were never broken.

You are simply built to notice more. And now, you are finally learning how to live well with all that you notice.

May that knowing carry you into a gentler future.

Printed in Dunstable, United Kingdom